Holistic Mental Health & Wellness:

The Complete Guide for Identifying and Treating the Physiological Contributors to Mental Health Symptoms

Niloo Dardashti PSYD HHP

ISBN: 1502856131
ISBN 13: 9781502856135
Library of Congress Control Number: 2014918688
CreateSpace Independent Publishing Platform
North Charleston, South Carolina

TABLE OF CONTENTS

INTRODUCTION

This is a general guide for people to follow when trying to help themselves achieve the mental wellness that they are entitled to. Think of it as a step by step manualized method for going down the path of identifying and treating the possible causes of your mental health symptoms.

As most of us know, the mind and body are integrally linked and often what affects one affects the other. However, the focus of this guide is on holistic MENTAL health wellness and I encourage you to run any suggestions you choose to follow by your physician first (hopefully one that gives you proper time/attention, and one you trust).

I created this manual because in working with my patients I realized there are so many layers to addressing mental health from a physiological standpoint and there needed to be an organized, systematic manual to do so. So, please be advised that this particular manual does not take into account the incredible impact of the psycho-emotional aspects to our mental health – including our relationships and the experiences we have had that have shaped us. Awareness of these aspects, in addition to awareness of our internal worlds, thoughts, and feelings are integral parts of achieving wellness and their importance should not be minimized. This guide, therefore, is a systematized way of identifying the *physiological* variables that play a role in how we feel and should not be assumed to be the sole contributors to why we feel depressed, anxious, etc. Instead, I invite you to think of it as one part – a baseline, if you will, for optimal functioning. In my experience, if you can get your baseline functioning to where it can be, the work you do on your self and your relationships can be a whole lot more fruitful.

The best way that you can use the information provided in this guide is to think about your "symptoms" long term – at least in the last year. Do some of these issues seem to have been present for you in the last year? Do you have a healthcare provider that you feel safe with who you might discuss some of these possibilities with, without feeling judged or rushed? This is very important as some of the diagnostic tests will require a willing doctor to help get answers.

Now without further ado, let's begin.

Part I:

The Role of Diet

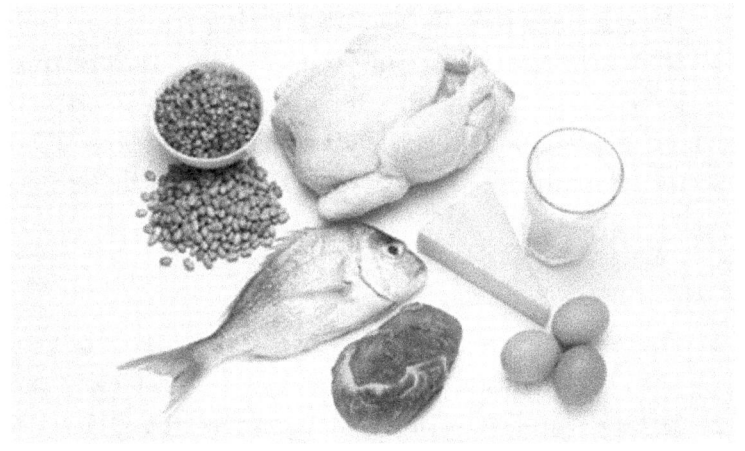

1. The Food-Mood Connection

Many individuals are not aware of how different foods affect their moods and overall feelings of well-being. How do you feel when you eat French fries as opposed to a salad? How do you feel when you eat fruit as opposed to a bag of doritos? Which foods seem to "drain" your energy the most? If you have never truly paid attention to your particular food-mood connection, your first step is to start keeping a log of what you eat on a daily basis with a rating scale (say 1-10, 10 being feeling best) and start keeping track of this. Food is literally the fuel for life and, knowing which foods affect us in certain ways, it is entirely possible to functionally use food as medicine.

2. Carbs Versus Protein

There is no question that we live in a carb-focused society. Bread, pasta, potatoes, and sugar are a few of the carb-heavy parts of most of our diets as Americans. The problem is that along with a multitude of other concerns, carbs create blood sugar surges that are detrimental to mental health. This is not to say that carbs should be avoided at all costs or that this is an all-or-nothing concept. For one thing there are good carbs, and not so good carbs; but one must know that that protein is literally fuel for neurotransmitters – the substances in one's brain that strongly impacts one's mental health status. In my opinion, vegetarians who choose to be vegetarian because they think it is healthier often run up against major roadblocks and frequently do not feel very well. It is challenging to get all the protein we need from just vegetarian sources. Here are some great sources of protein. Since many people with mental health symptoms are sensitive to dairy I have included only two examples of dairy products:

- Organic chicken and turkey
- Organic eggs
- Wild Alaskan Salmon
- If you choose tuna, go with chunklight skipjack, which has the least mercury in it
- Greek yogurt (if dairy tolerant)
- Organic cottage cheese (if dairy tolerant)
- RAW nuts and seeds
- Organic lentils
- Organic Black Rice
- Grassfed beef, lamb, and pork (in moderation)
- Whey Protein Concentrate from Grassfed sources, no sugar added (technically dairy but many dairy-intolerant folks do fine with it)
- Brown Rice protein
- Quinoa
- I always prefer to make my own shakes but if I'm on-the-go I like Orgain protein shakes

3. The Role of good fats

Good fats are necessary for many integral biochemical conversions. One must not forget about this very important aspect of our diets. For instance, often those individuals who are not getting enough omega three's show symptoms of depression, inattentiveness, and/or anxiety. "Good" fats are integral for proper brain function. Some examples of good fats are:

- Coconut oil
- Fish oils
- Flaxseed oil
- Real butter
- Olive oil
- Avocados

4. Food Toxins linked to mental health symptoms

- Saccharine
- Aspartame breaks down to formaldehyde (excitotoxin)
- "Excitotoxicity" is the pathological process by which <u>nerve cells</u> are damaged and killed by glutamate and similar substances. This has been said to be implicated in pain, fatigue, depression, anxiety, insomnia and other issues

Excitotoxins

- MSG – some people are quite sensitive to this substance
- Hydrolysed Protein – flavor enhancer
- Caseinate – flavor enhancer
- Autolyzed Yeast – flavor enhancer
- Carrageenan – thickening agent
- Aspartame (Nutrasweet/Equal)

5. **Mental Health Supporting Diet**
   The following are my general recommendations pertaining to protein and carb intake.

   - Eat protein three or more times a day. Try to include vegetables as the source of carbs with each meal. If you'd like a starch, choose black or brown rice, or quinoa. Include fruits (such as blueberries) and raw nuts as snacks in between meals.
   - I never preach to avoid sugar all together. Part of the quality of life is to enjoy certain foods and unless you have a severe intolerance or reaction to sugar, I think it is totally fine to have a (small) sweet every day. Eat it mindfully, in moderation, use it as a reward, and most importantly don't give yourself sh*t afterwards for eating it! Some examples of sweets to choose from are:
     - Ginny's gluten and dairy free organic chocolate chip cookies (they're good, believe me!)
     - Organic dark chocolate
     - A small amount of organic ice cream with almond or coconut milk if you are dairy intolerant
     - In general: look for amount of sugar per serving to be around 10 grams or less if possible
   - Drink lots of water. You probably hear this all the time, but it is important to remember because often when people feel lack of energy it is due at least in part to dehydration.

In addition, please keep in mind: *When you do not get enough protein in your diet, it can affect the vacillations of blood sugar.*

6. What are some possible symptoms of Blood Sugar issues?

HYPOGLYCEMIA

- Impatient, moody, nervous

- Crave sweets, starches, or alcohol

- Wake up in middle of night craving sweets

- Poor concentration, confusion, forgetfulness

- Irritable, tired, or weak if meal is missed

- Heart palpitations after eating sweets

- Feel tired 1 – 3 hours after eating

- Dizziness when standing suddenly

- Calmer after eating

HYPERGLYCEMIA

- Sugar in urine

- Depression

- Night sweats

- Increased thirst

- Family history of diabetes

- Fatigue

- Boils and leg sores

- Lesions, cuts take a long time to heal

- Overweight

As you can see, blood sugar problems can account for many mental health symptoms. In order to rule this out, Glucose Tolerance Testing would be a good idea. This includes: Glycohemoglobin and fasting and post prandial measures of glucose and insulin.

Nutrients That Level Blood Sugar
- Glutamine, 500 mg (1-3) x 3-4, chromium 400 mcg x 2-3
- Blood Sugar-Supportive Multi w/chromium, biotin, B complex
- Cinnamon
- PROTEIN

7. Gluten and Dairy

- If gluten and/or dairy is a significant factor for you (in terms of mental health symptoms), a two week trial of removal will tell a lot. We now know that inflammation is correlated with depression. Gluten can cause inflammation. Sometimes blood tests do not show sensitivities to gluten or dairy but people still feel much better when they take one or both of these out of their diets. The only way to know is to do the trial removal. A one month trial is best but two weeks is better than nothing
- Foods to avoid if you are going gluten free: gluten grains: barley, bulgar, kamut, oats, rye, spelt, white flour, wheat, semolina, couscous, durum flour, vital wheat gluten, commercial pasta, bagels, bread, muffins, and any ready to

eat cereal or any foods that contain any of these grains. In addition: processed meats, soy burgers and other "mock" meats, malt, barley malt, modified food starch, many alcoholic beverages – such as beer, and whiskey. In general, look for "gluten free"

- Non gluten grain choices include: amaranth, brown rice, buckwheat, millet, teff, quinoa, breads and ready to eat cereals made from these grains. Legume choices: adzuki, black eye peas, black turtle beans, garbanzo beans, kidney beans, lentils, lima beans, mung beans, navy beans, peas, pinto beans. Also, check out http://www.glutenfreeinfo.com/diet/glutenfreeinfo.htm

- Food sensitivities sometimes play a role in mental health symptoms. There are two types of allergies: IgE and IgG. IgE allergies are probably what you normally hear about in terms of an immediate, often very acute, reaction. IgG allergies exhibit more of a delayed reaction and can often be missed when doctors only check IgE allergies. ALCAT labs are great for testing both IgE and IgG allergies and you can discuss this with your doctor. Often only integrative docs will do this type of testing but it is good to be informed and you can certainly inform your doctor! Once you find out what food allergies may be contributing to symptoms you can remove those foods and help your digestion with probiotics.

- Probiotics are essential for healthy gut flora. We now know that there is a strong gut-brain connection and that probiotics can often help all sorts of mental health symptoms. It is also good to switch up your probiotics once in a while. Some examples of probiotics that I recommend are:
  - Garden of Life Primal Defense Ultra
  - Innate Response Formulas Flora 50-14 Clinical Strength
  - Essential Formulas Dr. Ohhira's Probiotics

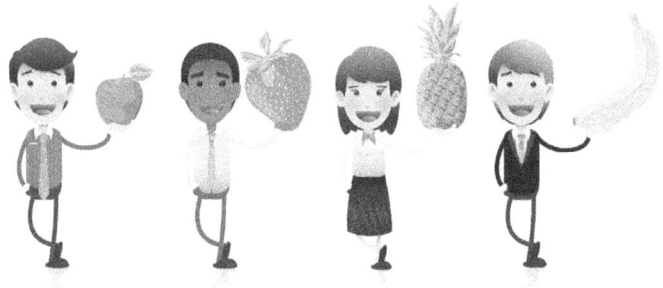

Part II:

Nutrient Depletion & Biochemistry Testing

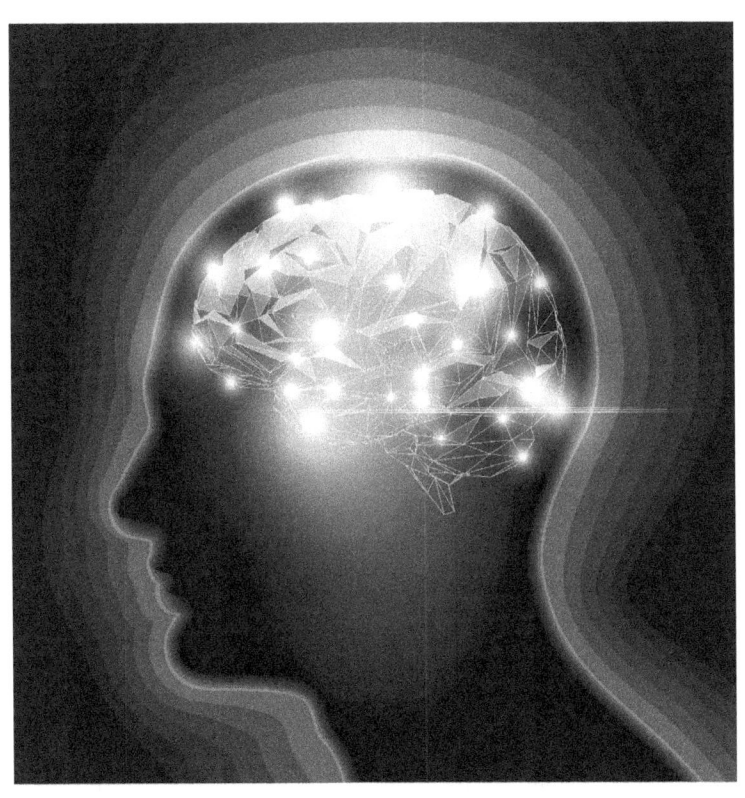

<u>Nutrition and Mental Health</u>

1. Some of the pioneers in the subject of orthomolecular psychiatry (nutrition and mental health) are Abram Hoffer, MD and Carl Pfeiffer, PhD, MD, Linus Pauling, PhD. I suggest getting acquainted with their work if this topic is strongly of interest for you.

2. Vitamins and minerals are important cofactors involved in neurotransmitter functioning. Sometimes we are deficient in one or many of these nutrients and this can be attributed to diet, personal metabolism, genetics, or lack of exposure to them. Though many people eat well, unfortunately our soils are depleted in a large number of nutrients and we are often not getting adequate amounts of them despite efforts to eat well. I highly recommend starting to research the companies, farms, and restaurants that your food choices come from to see what their standards and practices are. However, most people will find that they feel better with some supplementation in addition to their well-balanced diets. In the appendix, you will find a list of food sources for the various vitamins and minerals needed in our diets.

3. I also recommend eating organic as much as possible and especially to look for non-GMO (genetically modified) foods. When a food is organic, it is by default going to be non-GMO. Films such as Food Inc are great resources for explaining the GMO problem in our country. Foods that I highly recommend organic:

    o "The dirty dozen" as listed by the Environmental Working Group (apples, strawberries, grapes, celery, peaches, spinach,

> sweet bell peppers, imported nectarines, cucumbers, cherry tomatoes, imported snap peas and potatoes) See http://www.ewg.org/ for a variety of helpful resources
> o Meat products
> o Dairy products
> o Corn, soy, vegetable oils, and potatoes should be non-GMO. They are in almost everything!

4. BIOCHEMICAL TESTING CAN HELP

If you have symptoms and standard blood tests don't seem to come up with much, Genova and Spectracell laboratories are great labs for doing functional biochemistry testing. Ask your doctor about opening an account with spectracell for (at least) nutritional testing and Genova for (at least) Organic Acid testing. I find these can be very helpful in understanding what may be going on under the surface in terms of nutrient depletion and needs for particular cofactors. In the appendix, there is a list of vitamins and mineral depletions that correlate with symptoms as indicated by Spectracell Labs. Additionally, Neuroscience Lab provides urinary neurotransmitter and salivary adrenal testing, which can be very helpful in figuring out the cause of symptoms as well. In general I always say to people: "You are your best advocate." Start out with asking your doctor to do a bloodtest for the following mental health related nutrient & hormone levels, in addition to food allergy and methylation tests:

B12, folate, B6 carnitine, vitamin d (should be around 50), zinc, copper, selenium, magnesium, co-q10, iron, ferritin (should be at least 50 – implicated in ADHD, Restless Legs Syndrome), blood sugar (specifically glycohemoglobin A1C, and, if blood sugar issue is suspected, fasting and post prandial measures of glucose and insulin), full thyroid (including TSH, free T3, total T4, reverse T3, TPO antibodies), dhea, full hormone panel (during luteal phase for women – days 18 to 21 of the cycle), prolactin, iodine (sometimes correlated with thyroid proglems and better to check through urine), gluten and casein sensitivity, IgA and IgG/IgE blood tests for food allergies, heavy metal testing if suspected (especially if you have amalgam fillings or eat a lot of tuna), homocysteine and methylmalonic acid (high levels can indicate problems with methylation), and MTHF-R mutation (blood test).

When you receive the results of your bloodwork, always ask your physician for copy and look through the results with him/her so you can be well informed about what the different values mean. If you have a "borderline" number, this may mean you tested on the low end of that nutrient and perhaps supplementing with it can help even though you are not "deficient" per se. Discuss the idea of supplementing if this is the case. Once again, you are always your best advocate.

5. What is METHYLATION?

According to Mark Hyman, a well-respected integrative physician, it is a "key biochemical process that is essential for the proper function of almost all of your body's systems. It occurs billions of times every second; it helps repair your DNA on a daily basis; it controls homocysteine (an unhealthy compound that can damage blood vessels); it helps recycle molecules needed for detoxification; and it helps maintain mood and keep inflammation in check."

Proper methylation depends on several b vitamins – most importantly, b12, folate, and b6. If you find out that you have an issue with methylation, Designs for Health makes a good product for homocysteine/methylation support called Homocysteine Support.

6. What is an MTHF-R GENE MUTATION?

According to the National Institute of Health:
"What is the normal function of the *MTHFR* gene?
The *MTHFR* gene provides instructions for making an enzyme called methylenetetrahydrofolate reductase. This enzyme plays a role in processing amino acids, the building blocks of proteins. Methylenetetrahydrofolate reductase is important for a chemical reaction involving forms of the B-vitamin folate (also called folic acid or vitamin B9). Specifically, this enzyme converts 5,10-methylenetetrahydrofolate to 5-methyltetrahydrofolate. This reaction is required for the multistep process that converts the amino acid homocysteine to another amino acid, methionine. The body uses methionine to make proteins and other important compounds."

Adequate methylation is sometimes difficult because the body has a harder time creating a powerful detox substance called glutathione, so there is often an accumulation of toxins

- Treating this mutation with the most potent form of folate (5-methyltetrahydrafolate) can make a world of difference for these folks, many of whom suffer with depression or bipolar disorder. Metagenics makes a great one and you can find them all over now. Metafolin and deplin are prescription strength doses.
- Sam-E can be very helpful but do not use this if you have ever been diagnosed with or suspect you may be bipolar or even cyclothymic (a less intense form of bipolar disorder).

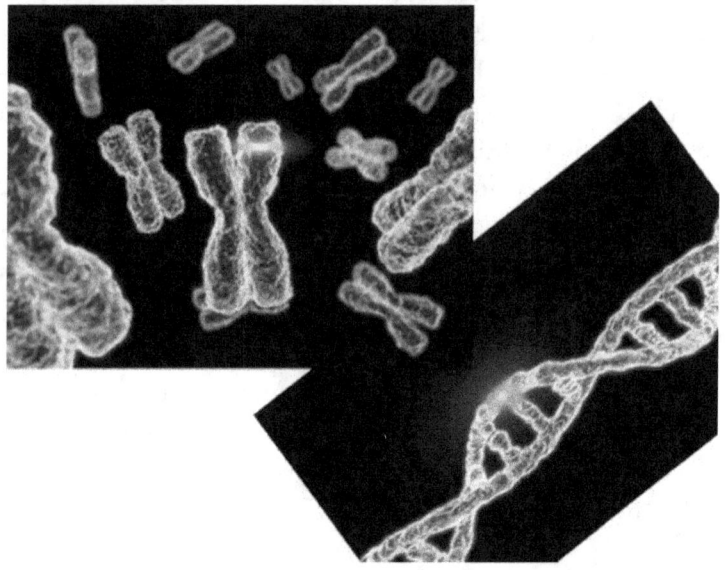

7. OTHER HELPFUL NUTRIENTS FOR MENTAL HEALTH: NAC

NAC (N-Acetylcysteine) is an amino acid precursor to glutathione. As mentioned, glutathione is involved in detoxification. NAC is used for many psychiatric conditions successfully; evidence based studies for its use in trichotillomania, OCD, and bipolar disorder have shown improvement in symptoms. Generally dosages start at 500 mg and go up to 3000 mg daily

8. OTHER HELPFUL NUTRIENTS FOR MENTAL HEALTH: INOSITOL

Inositol is a b vitamin that has good evidence for the treatment of OCD. One study using 18 grams of the powder improved symptoms significantly

9. ....IN ADDITION

Epsom salt baths are a great way to get magnesium and have a wonderful calming effect on anxiety, in addition to helping sore muscles – one cup in a warm bath for ½ hour will do wonders.

10. Zinc / Copper Balance

The issue of zinc /copper balance is a cornerstone of orthomolecular psychiatry. In general, we like to see equal amounts of these. When one has a high copper to zinc ratio we often see anxiety as a main symptom. Low copper on the other hand, is often correlated with difficulty concentrating. In my practice I see a lot more low zinc levels than copper. Often treating this issue can be extremely helpful.

11. OMEGA Three and Six Fatty Acids

There are plenty of studies implicating omega 3's in mood, attention, and a host of other issues. In general, we get much more omega six's in our foods than three's. Omega six fatty acids increase inflammation and are found in vegetable oils, (which many of our foods are comprised of). Therefore, in my opinion, it most important to focus on the crucial omega three's that many of us our low in. Specifically, we want a nice balance of EPA and DHA (the fatty acids that comprise fish oils). Eating more fish such as wild Alaskan salmon is also a great way to get omega three's. In terms of supplementation, two grams seems to be the starting active dose and also helps with inflammation, which is linked to mental health symptoms. Look for molecularly distilled brands, which focus on removing mercury from their fish oils.

12. A WORD ON INFLAMMATION

Inflammation is a major problem in our country and has been linked to depression and other mental health symptoms. In addition to an anti-inflammatory diet and fish oil, turmeric is one of the best natural anti-inflammatories. A recent study discussed in Life Extension magazine reported that 500 mg administered twice per day helped depressed patients just as much as Prozac. This is incredible.

Other effective natural anti-inflammatories include: bromelein (an enzyme found in pineapples), bosweila (an herb), and Zyflamend (a product made by New Chapter, which contains a variety of herbs).

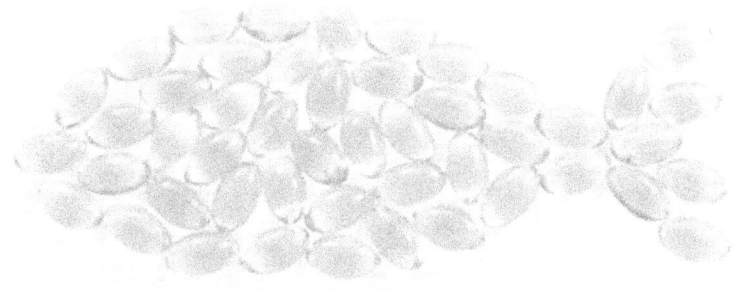

Part III:

Targeted Amino Acid Therapy

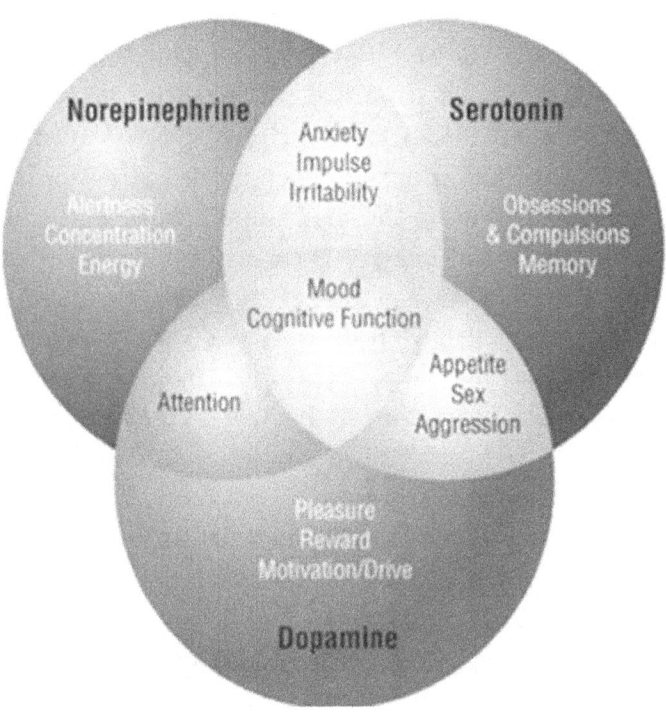

1. Amino acids are the building blocks to our neurotransmitters. When we think about neurotransmitters we generally want to thinking about them as "excitatory" or "inhibitory." **Excitatory neurotransmitters** are those that make us stimulated and help with focus, mood, and attention. They are also called "catecholamines" and include epinephrine, norepinephrine, and dopamine. **Inhibitory neurotransmitters** play a role in helping us to feel calm and regulating mood. They include serotonin and gaba. When deciding which amino acids may be helpful, one can think about symptoms that have to do with low (or high) levels of the neurotransmitters listed above. As discussed in the previous section, Neuroscience Lab does urinary neurotransmitter testing to help indicate which amino acids could be helpful; however, there is some controversy about whether these tests are truly accurate. I do not see any harm in taking the test (along with a salivary cortisol test, I have found it to be very helpful) but often it is possible to try aminos based on the particular symptoms one is having. In her book "The Mood Cure," Julia Ross goes into great detail regarding this matter. I recommend her book. Below, I have given examples of symptoms relating to depletions in the neurotransmitters discussed.

<u>Symptoms of Low Serotonin may include:</u>

- Depressed mood, often accompanied by agitation or irritability

- Anxiety or panic
- Restlessness and quick to anger
- Obsessive thoughts or behaviors
- Problems sleeping
- Carb and/or sugar cravings

<u>Symptoms of Low GABA may include:</u>

- General widespread sense of tension or unease
- Anxiety that presents as over stimulation or "wired"
- Stressed and burnt out
- Craving substances for relaxing because of an inability to do so
- Trouble sleeping

<u>Symptoms of Low Catecholamines may include:</u>

- Depressed mood accompanied by apathy and/or lethargy
- Lack of energy, focus, motivation and/or follow-through
- Difficulty experiencing pleasure
- Cravings for stimulation from substances such as caffeine, chocolate, methamphetamines, cocaine, Ritalin, marijuana

2. Amino Acid Dosing

- Aminos should be taken 1/2 hour before or 2 hours after protein with water or juice

- It takes about 20-30 minutes for aminos to get into the system
- In general changes can be expected in 1-3 weeks
- Start with the lowest dose possible and go up slowly until you notice change Children should be closely monitored by a physician
- Stop if you notice any adverse reaction
- Reassess after 1-2 months; dosing should not be ongoing indefinitely
- **General dosing strategy: 500 – 1500 mg 1-3 x daily. (5htp equivalent is 50-150 mg).** In my experience, people usually take aminos twice per day

<u>Serotonin Boosting Amino Acids</u>

- Start with 5HTP (50 mg). Some even start with 25 mg chewables. If you know you have high cortisol or you have insomnia, choose L-tryptophan instead. Both of these amino acids help with serotonin building. But choose one OR the other
- Tryptophan→5HTP→Serotonin→Melatonin
- 5HTP is better when one is also fatigued since it can have a small cortisol raising effect
- Use caution with: bipolar spectrum tendencies, severe or suicidal depression, carcinoid tumor, asthma, excessively high cortisol output (5HTP)
- Contraindications: Ischemic heart disease (e.g., a history of myocardial infarction, angina pectoris or documented silent ischemia), coronary artery

spasm (e.g., Prinzmetal sangina), uncontrolled hypertension or any other significant cardiovascular disease. Talk to your doctor.

- Speak to your physician if you are taking any serotonergic drugs such as SSRI's, naratriptan, sumatriptan and zolmitriptan.

Catecholamine Boosting Amino Acids

- L-Tyrosine or L-phenylalanine 500-1500 mg 2-3 times per day
- Make sure to take only in the morning and during the earlier part of the day as these aminos can be stimulating
- Some people do better with one or the other of the above. True Focus by Now has both and some people really like this product
- EPA/DHA can also help with this
- If you have pain or mood issues as well, DL-Phenylalinine (DLPA) might be worth a try
- Contraindications: Overactive thyroid (Grave's disease), PKU (phenylketonuria)
- Use caution with: high blood pressure, migraine headaches, bipolar spectrum tendencies, Hashimoto's

GABA Boosting Amino Acids

- GABA 100-500 mg and/or 1-4 times per day OR kavinace 1-3 times per day. Kavinace is a product by Neuroscience lab which many of my patients do very well with. It is mostly a combination of phenylbutyric acid (a derivative of GABA) and taurine (an amino acid that helps facilitate production of GABA)

- Pharma Gaba is a chewable supplement that is sometimes more easily absorbed than Gaba on its own. Natural Factors makes a version that many of my patients do very well with
- L-Theanine (at least 100 mg) generally 200-800 mg per day
    o Theanine raises both gaba and dopamine so it helps with alertness as well as anxiety. It enhances the alpha brain state
- Use caution with: very low blood pressure

Symptoms of Low Endorphin

- In addition to the neurotransmitter depletions that people often have, it is also possible to have low levels of endorphins. People with this issue often are very sensitive to emotional (or physical) pain, cry easily, often feel "numb," and/or crave pleasure, comfort, and reward.
- This may present in the form of addiction and substance abuse

Boosting Endorphin Levels

- D-phenylalinine (DPA) 500-1000 mg 1-3 times per day. If attention, focus and energy are also an issue, DL-Phenylalanine (DLPA) can be tried

- Genesa makes a product called Complete Free Form Amino Blend and provides dosing strategies on its website
- Acupuncture and cranial osteopathy can also help
- What is the reason for underlying pain? This is important to find out. In some cases a person could have undiagnosed lyme, fibromyalgia, and/or some structural issue

Compulsive and/or emotional eating

Some people have food "addictions" or compulsive eating problems as part of their low neurotransmitter symptoms

- In general:
  - o Use 5HTP or L-tryptophan to raise serotonin for afternoon and evening cravings – especially pertaining to sugar and carb cravings
  - o L-glutamine and chromium can help with cravings in addition to regulating blood sugar. Take these in the morning as they can be stimulating. Also, avoid L-glutamine if you have bipolar spectrum tendencies or if you have ever had lymphatic cancer
  - o Use dosing strategies for DLPA to raise endorphins for comfort food cravings and foods craved for energy boosts (am and/or mid-morning as this can be stimulating)

o   Try Pharma Gaba if you are eating to calm
    yourself down when stressed
o   Speak to your doctor before starting any
    course of amino acids

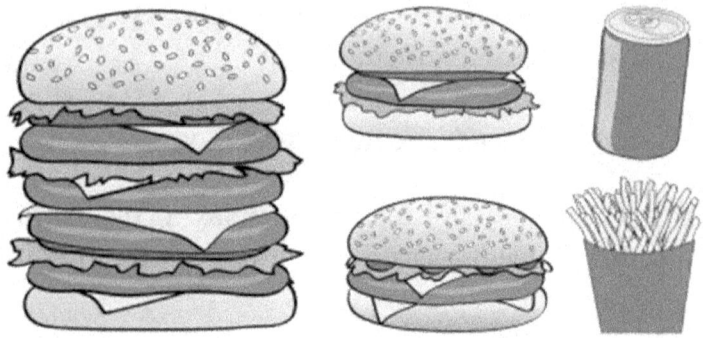

Part IV:

Holistic Strategies for Treating ADHD

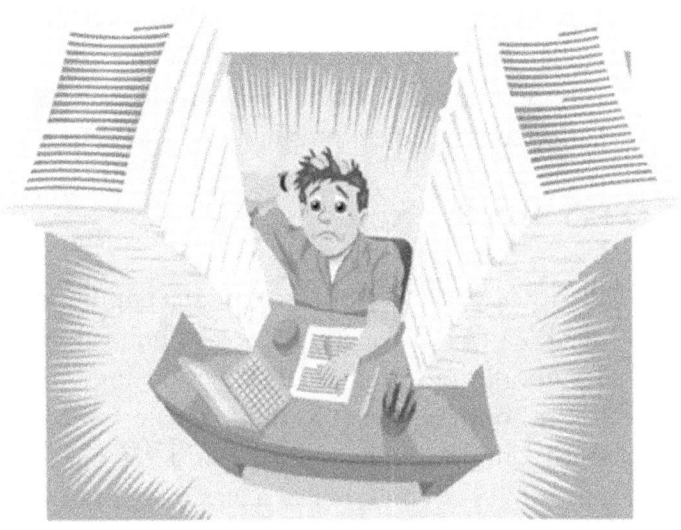

1. AMINO ACIDS

- Many people with ADD or ADHD have low levels of catecholamines such as norepinephrine and/or dopamine. For this reason, it is best to think about trying the amino acid l-tyrosine or l-phenylalinine
- Start with tyrosine because l-phenylalinine takes longer for conversion
- True Focus by Now has both and many of my patients have found it helpful. Some individuals are very sensitive to these amino acids and Neuroscience makes a product called Clari-T which is a chewable l-tyrosine with only 250 mg per tablet
- If restlessness and hyperactivity are an issue, 5HTP, gaba, kavinace, or tryptophan can also help

2. FATTY ACIDS

- Plenty of research concludes that a combination of EPA and DHA seems to be very helpful. About 1 g per day of EPA and DHA is a starting point
- Phosphotidylserine (PS) did better in one study, but it was only tested against 250 mg of fish oil. PS is a member of a class of chemical compounds known as *phospholipids*. It is an essential component in all our cells, specifically the cell membrane. In addition to learning and attention, PS is also great for memory
- Best seems to be combo of both (PS and fish oil)

3. SAM-E & HERBAL STIMULANTS

- SAM-E: B12 or folate deficiency = lower levels of SAM-E, which can add to and facilitate ADD symptoms, particularly inattentive types. SAM-E should be taken on an empty stomach but should be avoided in people with bipolar disorder or people who have a lot of anxiety
- 200-1000 mg of B12 can also help and should also be avoided in anxious or bipolar people unless one knows of a deficiency. Go slow
- Herbal stimulants: pycnogenol, gingko, ginseng. Pycnogenol seems to have the best conclusive evidence for being helpful with ADHD – particularly the restless type

4. OTHER CONSIDERATIONS

- Try to reduce electronic stimulation
- Time Management Reinforcement for perceived self-efficacy
  - o Pomodoro Technique helps with this: Check out http://pomodorotechnique.com/
- Mindfulness training – see the appendix for a more detailed explanation. Mindfulness has been proven to be helpful for a plethora of issues, from depression to anxiety to chronic pain and anger management. I believe it is an integral part to getting a handle on most mental health symptoms.

Part V:

Holistic Strategies for Treating Insomnia

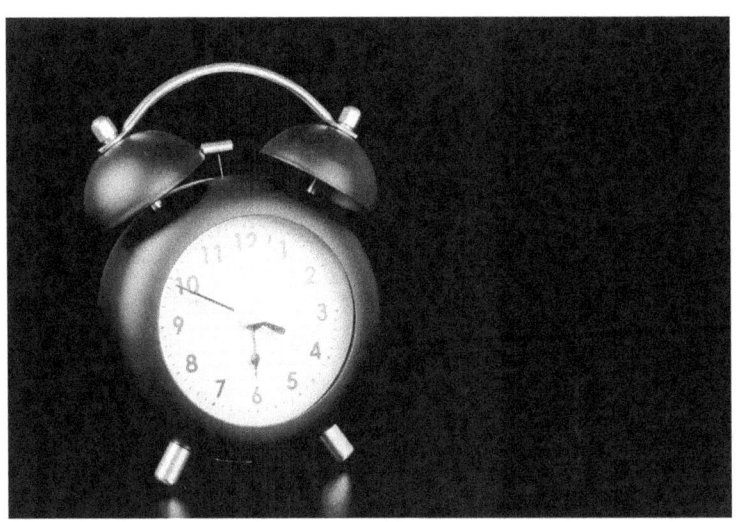

1. There are many different manifestations of sleep disturbance. The first one is what most people think of when they hear the word "insomnia." This type is characterized by not being able to get to sleep in the first place and many of these people report that they cannot turn off their minds. This is often due to low melatonin and serotonin levels. Treatment:

   - L-Tryptophan (500 mg-1500 mg) or 5HTP (50 mg-150 mg) by 10 PM. Both of these help with conversion of serotonin to melatonin. Start with 500 mg of tryptophan (or 50 mg 5HTP) on the first night. Go up to 3 caps (1500 mg tryptophan or 150 mg 5HTP) by the third night if the first two dosages don't help.
     - If after the third night you find that the increased dosage did not work, add melatonin immediate release 1-3 mg or melatonin two-stage release 1-3 mg, for those who also have later insomnia
     - Most people with insomnia do better with tryptophan since 5HTP has a small cortisol raising effect
   - For those who feel that they are too tense or stressed to sleep, gaba may be more appropriate as they may be low in this neurotransmitter. Treatment:
     - GABA 100-500 mg and/or Taurine OR kavinace

2. For those people who wake up between 2-5 AM (or earlier,) and feel like they are ready to jump out of

bed, there may be an issue with elevated cortisol at night. Treatment:

- Test salivary cortisol levels and/or provide a cortisol lowering substance called phosphorylated serine. This is a more active form of phosphatidylserine and is sold under the name "seriphos." It should not be taken for more than about a month at a time. It is best to measure cortisol levels at baseline and then measure again after taking seriphos. Also, by measuring cortisol, it is easier to see what time of night it would be best to take the seriphos dose

3. Other important contributors to sleep disturbance

- Sleep Apnea, Upper Airway Resistance, other sleep-breathing problems. If this is suspected, a sleep study is in order
- Lighting in the bedroom is crucial. Even the light emanating from your alarm clock can affect you if you have trouble with melatonin production. The message to the pineal gland (where melatonin is made) must be loud and clear: it is nighttime and time to go to sleep. Therefore, black out drapes are a great idea as are special amber light bulbs for nighttime purposes (such as reading in bed before going to sleep)
- High glutamate levels. Blue lights (the ones that are all around us in our lighting and screens), inhibit melatonin – they also activate glutamate,

an excitatory neurotransmitter that some of us are very sensitive to

- Therefore, in addition to optimal lighting in the bedroom, dim all lights by 7 pm, restrict ANY screen exposure 2 hours before bed, and use amber-hue lights. Resources: LowBlueLights. com, f.lux. If a neuroscience test finds that you have high glutamate levels, you can also take l-theanine, which is said to reduce glutamate
- Restless Legs Syndrome and Periodic Limb Movement Disorder. Dopamine related and linked to levels of Ferritin below 50
- Partner moving around in bed. I often suggest that couples get a king frame and put two twin extra-long mattresses in it. Even subtle stimulation can affect the quality of your sleep
- Supplements or meds taken at night. Many people tell me they have sleep problems and during a thorough evaluation I find that they are taking some of their vitamins at night. Many vitamins have slight or strong stimulating effects and especially people with sleep issues can be very sensitive to these. For example, biotin, a b vitamin that many women take for their hair, can be stimulating. If you are concerned, try taking your vitamins with breakfast and do some research
- To-do list. If your mind is racing with all the things you need to do, creating a to-do list and keeping it by your bedside can help. Feeling like you need to remember something and being

worried that you won't can disrupt your ability to relax enough to get to sleep

- Dr. Weil's 4-7-8 breath. This has been proven to help people wind down. Inhale for a count of 4 seconds, hold for 7 seconds, and exhale for a count of 8 seconds
- Brown noise machines for low frequency noises. Many people use noise machines to help with blocking noises, which I highly encourage. Interestingly, most noise machines supply "white noise," whereas some supply "brown noise," a noise frequency that is supposed to help block out more low-frequency sounds which are harder to block out with white noise
- Avoid eating a couple hours before bedtime. If you get very hungry, try having a few raw almonds. They have magnesium in them which is calming and the protein can help with stabilizing your blood sugar. This is especially a good choice for those who wake up with spiking blood sugar levels. Some people do better with a light carb snack before bed. Experiment to see what is right for you
- Circadian Rhythm Disturbance
  - o To reset: wake up with an alarm clock between 6 and 7 am, sit outside in the sunshine, stay awake and wait until 9 or 10 PM to sleep (for at least 2 to 3 days in a row)
- Temperature Reduction and Optimization. A slight lowering of body temperature, which occurs at night, plays a very important role in

moderating the chemical signals that play a role in sleep induction
- Take an epsom salt bath a couple hours before bedtime. I have had patients tell me that this was an amazing antidote to their insomnia. This may be due to the absorption of magnesium, which is highly prevalent in Epsom salts

A word on Fatigue: "Fatigue" during the day may also be due to:
- Vitamin D Deficiency: levels should be between 50-70 mg/ml
- Carnitine Deficiency—A trial of 2 to 3 grams per day for a minimum of 6 to 8 weeks can be helpful
- Ribose Deficiency—5 grams 3 times daily significantly reduced fatigue in CFS patients

Part VI:

Adrenal Function and Mental Health Symptoms

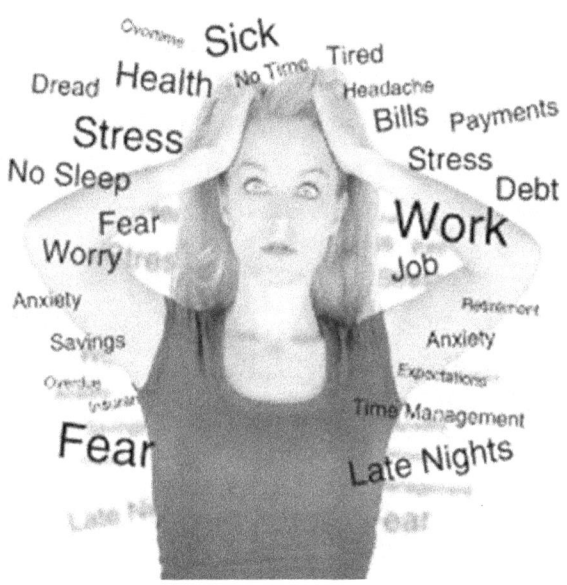

1. The main function of your adrenal glands (located at the top of your kidneys) is to help your body deal with any source of stressors – be they physical, environmental, or emotional. Your adrenals secrete cortisol, levels of which, as discussed above, can sometimes become imbalanced – either too high or too low (or both at different parts of the day). This is often due to a history of being under chronic stress.

2. Four point salivary cortisol testing can be very helpful in assessing adrenal issues.   Normally we like to see a robust cortisol in the morning that decreases by nighttime so one can settle down and get to sleep. With four point salivary testing, we can observe how the cortisol changes at four different times of the day – usually morning, mid-morning, afternoon, and evening. This can tell us if there is an adrenal problem playing a role in symptoms. Often this is part of the picture.

   Some high cortisol signs: Belly fat, inflammation, depression, PMS
   - **High Cortisol Treatment:** Schedule time to relax, limit caffeine & limit alcohol, consider L-theanine, Phosphatidylserine (PS), Omega 3's, Ashwaganha, Rhodiola, or Relora

   Some Low Cortisol Signs: Tired, burnt out, Difficulty fighting infection, Low BP
   - **Low Cortisol Treatment:** Exercise but don't overdue it, consider Vitamin C, Vitamins B1, B6,

B5, biotin, zinc, magnesium, Licorice, grapefruit juice if no SSRI's are being taken.

3. Adaptogens can help with regulating cortisol. According to the organization Life Extension, "adaptogens produce an increase in power of resistance against multiple stressors, including physical, chemical, or biological agents, normalize physiology, helping the body maintain youthful function, regardless of the cause of stress, normalize bodily functions beyond what is required to gain resistance to stress naturally, and exert a normalizing effect on cortisol."

4. In general, adaptogens should be taken for about 4-8 weeks, after which symptoms can be reassessed. Some examples of adaptogens are:
   - Rhodiola: about 150 mg 2-3 times daily. Also works on dopamine, norepinephrine, and serotonin. I prefer this if there is difficulty focusing too. This can sometimes increase anxiety so take it in the beginning of the day only.
   - Ashwagandha: I start with 125 mg and go up to 800 mg. This can sometimes increase anxiety so take in the beginning of the day only
   - Relora: (a combination of Magnolia bark extract and Phellodendron bark extract) helps some people get to sleep as well
   - Cortisol Manager by Integrative Therapeutics: a formula containing different nutrients that are designed to help with resistance to stress by balancing cortisol levels

5. DHEA is a hormone that is produced in the adrenal glands, gonads, brain, and skin. According to Life Extension, "In humans, DHEA is the dominant steroid hormone and precursor of all steroid sex hormones. Its role in sexual physiology (for both men and women) is that of a mood modulator. As we age, DHEA levels start to decline, so that by 70-80 years of age, peak DHEA concentrations are only 10-20% of those in young adults"

- Start slow and do baseline testing. Some women don't even need more than 5 mg daily. Only take it in the morning as it can be stimulating
- DHEA can be very helpful for mood and energy and can help ramp up adrenal functioning

6. Hypothyroidism

- **Symptoms:** Hair loss, dry skin, "thyroid hair", fatigue, weight gain, depression, cold hands/feet, constipation, cold intolerance
- **Diagnosis:** Work with your doctor to check TSH, T3, Free T3, T4, zinc, copper, mercury, vitamin D, selenium, iodine. Tyrosine is also a precursor and can be tried before starting meds
- There is much controversy on the issue of what is called "low T3 syndrome." Many people believe that taking T3 (cytomel) can help with subclinical and clinical hypothyroidism. T4 converts to T3 and the popular medicine synthroid is T4. Another option, Armour

Thyroid is derived from pigs and is a combination of T4 and T3. You can work with your doctor to figure out the best trial for you

- Depleted cortisol can lead to thyroid issues. Sometimes treating adrenal issues can thus help thyroid
- If T3 is low and is treated, antidepressant medications can often work better and vice versa

7. Hyperthyroidism

- **Symptoms:** nervousness or irritability, fatigue or muscle weakness, heat intolerance, trouble sleeping, hand tremors, rapid and irregular heartbeat, frequent bowel movements or diarrhea, weight loss, mood swings. Diagnosis is usually based on low levels of TSH. I see hypothyroidism much more often than hyperthyroidism.

Part VII:

Women's Health Conditions and Mental Health Symptoms

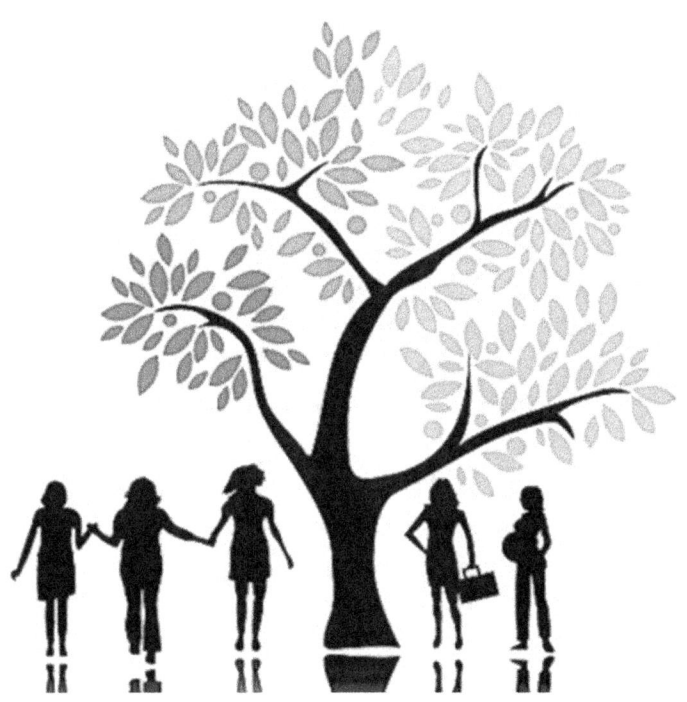

1. Estrogen Dominance: A condition in which the ratio of estrogen to progesterone is higher than it should be. Progesterone starts running out and women can have symptoms such as insomnia, mood swings and PMS, among many others. Think of progesterone as calming and estrogen as energizing.

2. Likewise, low estrogen can often be an issue and women often report symptoms such as depression, low libido, and low energy

3. PMS. Most women know how terrible it can feel to go through some spectrum of PMS symptoms. Some symptoms include irritability, cyclic headaches, irregular or heavy menses, and disrupted sleep.

   - PMS can often be due to low progesterone levels and therefore many women get much relief by using a progesterone cream
   - Getting this tested at baseline is very important as too much progesterone can make some women prone to depression
   - Serotonin and often gaba are also lower during the premenstrual time so some women feel better when supplementing with 5-HTP, tryptophan and/or gaba at this time

   ### Treatment for PMS:

   - Vitamin C
   - Chasteberry/vitex

- Calcium, magnesium, vitamin B1, 2, 6's, Vitamin D
- Omega 3's
- Evening primrose oil (omega 6)
- Exercise—frequency, not intensity—30 min 4x/week
- Acupuncture

4. PMDD (Premenstrual Dysphoric Disorder) is a much more severe form of PMS.
   - Women often report that they are suicidal or have paranoid thoughts
   - A combo of some natural therapies and/or a low dose SSRI can be very helpful

In helping women to identify how their cycles impact their moods and behaviors, I ask them to keep a chart/diary of the month for a few months. Day one is the first day of menstruation. We are generally looking for changes during menstruation, around ovulation, and during the luteal phase which is the period between ovulation and menstruation. Everyone is different and is impacted differently during different times of their cycle. I recommend Leslie Botha's book (Understanding Your Mind, Mood, and Hormone Cycle), which has an interesting take on changes in a woman's personality during her cycle

Part VIII:

Special Considerations

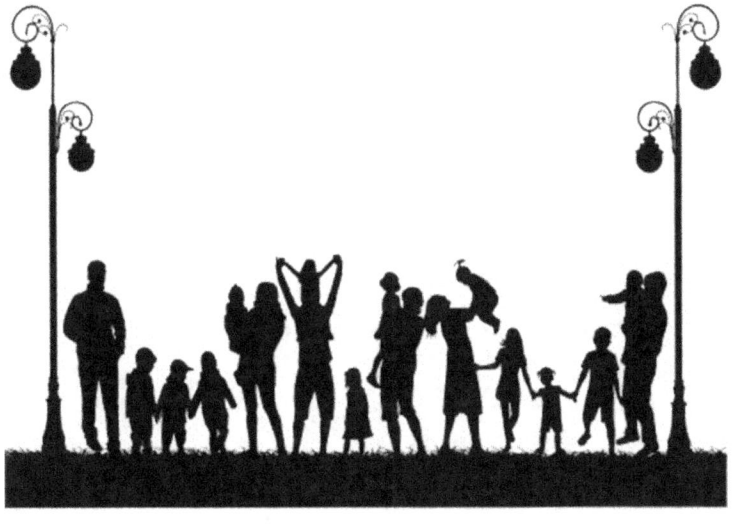

1. Seasonal Affective Disorder (SAD)

- **Symptoms:** depression, excessive sleeping, other sleep disturbances, carb cravings, social withdrawal. These symptoms seem to occur around the same time every year – usually the winter months.

Light Treatment

- o 7-9 AM is best
- o 10,000 lux is best for 30 min/day
- o Be 18 inches from light for all light boxes
- o Helps with circadian rebalancing
- o Vitamin D should be between 50-70

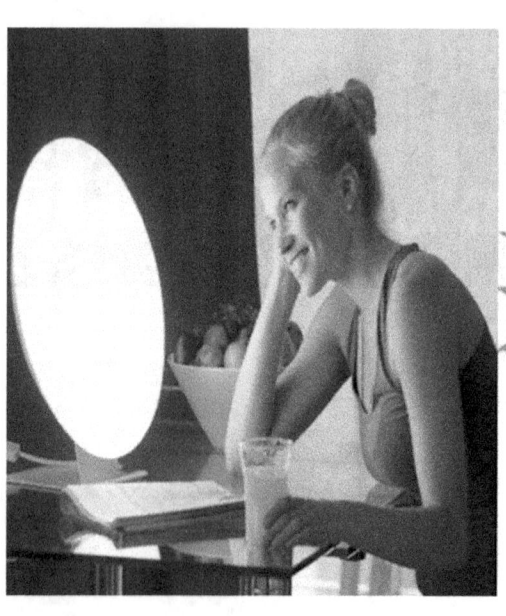
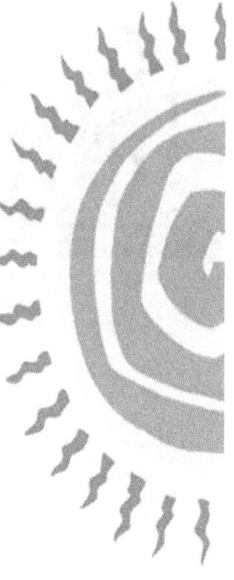

2. "Biotypes"

- According to Orthomolecular Psychiatry, there are specific "biotypes" that correlate with different mental health conditions. They are: Pyroluria, Histadelia, and Histapenia
- Eva Edelman's book "Natural Healing for Bipolar Disorder" describes these at length

3. Fungal Overgrowth and Candida

- Many practitioners strongly believe that these issues contribute to serious mental health symptoms (and subtle ones as well). We know that there is a significant connection between the gut and the brain so this is very likely in my opinion
- Candida is a controversial illness that is characterized by systemic yeast or fungal overgrowth. Many people with "candida" symptoms complain of "brain fog" as a primary symptom. Stool samples can be ordered through Genova or other labs to test for this, in addition to parasites, which can also affect mental health symptoms

4. Lyme Disease

- Often lyme and related co-infections are under diagnosed. In my opinion they may possibly be over diagnosed as well, with some physicians attributing symptoms entirely to borderline results. However, either way, with a positive lyme or co-infection result, there can be serious neurological and mental health symptoms.

- It is important to note that not everybody gets the bulls-eye mark which signals a bite
- Igenix lab seems to offer the most intensive testing for lyme at the present time
- If you suspect you may have been exposed at some point, try to see a lyme literate doctor. The Lyme Disease Association website is a good resource

5. Mercury Toxicity

- Another hot topic that is very controversial
- Dr. Andy Cutler has done extensive research on the effects of this on mental health symptoms
- Any heavy metal toxicity can exacerbate symptoms. Amalgam dental fillings, and high consumption of sushi / tuna are regular causes of high mercury levels. If you get your amalgams removed, make sure to undergo the process very carefully and look for a dentist who understands the risks of mercury poisoning. The International Academy of Oral Medicine & Toxicology website is a great resource and provides a directory of dentists

6. Exercise

- The benefits of exercise on mood are wide known. Often it is difficult to get started.

- I recommend the slow-burn method for 15 minutes twice per week to start. In general, as you start to notice changes, your feelings of self-efficacy will increase and therefore the behavior (in this case exercise) is likely to be reinforced. Check out http://en.wikipedia.org/wiki/Super_Slow

7. Breathing

- This is a simplistic but very important intervention. Most people breathe shallowly, from their chest rather than their diaphrams, or very little in general! You always have your breath. As soon as you become aware of it, focus on breathing correctly and you will notice subtle to significant changes in your physiological arousal. If you are really not in tune with your ability to deep breathe, take a pranayama class. This is the part of yoga that is just focused on using the breath

Some Helpful Resources

- Julia Ross – The Mood Cure
- Joan Mathews Larson, PhD – Depression-Free Naturally
- William Walsh, PhD –Nutrient Power
- Eva Edelman – Natural Healing for Bipolar Disorder

- Graceyln Guyol - Healing Depression & Bipolar Disorder Without Drugs: Inspiring Stories of Restoring Mental Health Through Natural Therapies
- Richard Brown – Rhodiola Revolution
- Environmental Working Group website
- American Association of Integrative Medicine website/directory
- International Network of Integrative Mental Health

APPENDIX

<u>**Vitamins in Food Sources according to BodyBio Inc**</u>

- Food sources of Vitamin A:
  - o Organic liver, dandelion greens, collard greens, sweet potato, beet greens, dried nonsulfured apricots, kale, sweet potato, parsley, spinach, butternut squash, mango, red pepper, cantaloupe, broccoli, papaya, eggs, cherries, asparagus, tomatoes, green peas, prunes
- Food sources of Thiamin/Vitamin B1:
  - o Turkey-dark meat, buckwheat, millet, brazil nuts, sesame seeds, potato flour, soybeans, eggplant, sunflower seeds, wheat germ, rice polishings, pine nuts, pork, pecans, slip peas, pistachio nuts, navy beans
- Food Sources of Riboflavin/Vitamin B2:
  - o Venison, clams, brewers yeast, organic liver and heart, Alaskan salmon, turkey,

pumpkin seeds, seaweed, soybeans, feta cheese, ricotta cheese, almonds, mushrooms, egg yolks, blueberries, buckwheat, wheat germ

- Food Sources of Niacin/Niacinemide/Vitamin B3:
  o Avocado, buckwheat, brown rice, clams, haddock, herring, mackerel, Alaskan salmon, organic beef, venison, chicken, Cornish game hen, duck, turkey, sesame seeds, sunflower seeds, soybeans, asparagus, lima beans, mushrooms, sweet potato
- Food Sources of Pyridoxine/Vitamin B6:
  o Avocado, casaba melon, brown rice, wheat germ, cod, shad, red snapper, beef, chicken, turkey, chestnuts, sunflower seeds, filberts, soybeans, walnuts, Alaskan salmon, lentils, lima beans, garbanzo beans, eggplant, hearts of palm, sweet potato
- Food Sources of Cobalamin (Vitamin B12):
  o Egg yolk, beef, organic beef liver, venison, chicken giblets, turkey giblets, clams, herring, lobster, Alaskan salmon, sardines, red snapper, trout
- Food Sources of Folic Acid:
  o Avocado, boysenberries, casaba melon, papaya, amaranth, buckwheat, rye, wheat germ, crab, shad roe, chicken, turkey, organic liver, cashew, filbert, pistachio nuts, pumpkin seeds, walnuts, artichoke, asparagus, lima beans, black beans, navy beans, pinto beans, mung sprouts, beets,

broccoli, bok choy, Chinese cabbage, mustard greens, black-eyed peas, green peas, seaweed, soybeans, spinach, kidney beans, lentils

- Food Sources of Biotin:
  - o Egg yolk, liver, walnuts, pecans, cottage cheese, goat cheese, mozzarella cheese, muenster cheese, ricotta cheese, yogurt, avocado, papaya, watermelon, dark rye flower, wheat germ, rice polishings, herring, lobster, mussels, flounder, organic liver, almonds, cashews, filberts, macadamia nuts, black-eyed peas, sweet potato
- Food Sources of Choline:
  - o Soy lecithin, egg yolk, wheat germ, black eyed peas, chick peas, brewer's yeast, lentils, split peas, asparagus, soybeans, rice polishings, organ meats, peanuts
- Food Sources of Inositol:
  - o Organ meats, soy lecithin, wheat germ, navy beans, rice polishings, brewer's yeast, black eyed peas, chick peas, orange, lima beans, green peas, lentil, cantaloupe, brown rice, peach, cabbage, cauliflower, onion
- Food Sources of Pantothenic Acid:
  - o Peanuts, mushrooms, split peas, brewer's yeast, organic liver, soybeans, pecans, eggs, lobster, buckwheat sunflower seeds, lentils
- Food Sources of Vitamin D:
  - o Eggs, herring, mackerel, oysters, Alaskan salmon, cod liver, shrimp, sunflower seeds, mushrooms

- Food Sources of Vitamin C:
    - o Blackberries, cantaloupe, black currants elderberries, gooseberries, grapefruit, guava, honeydew, melon, kiwi, orange, papaya, pineapple, raspberries, strawberries, tangerine, watermelon, fava beans, sweet red peppers, tomatoes, brussel sprouts, kale, broccoli
- Food Sources of Flavonoids:
    - o Apricots, blackberries, black currents, broccoli, cabbage, cantaloupe, cherries, grapefruit, grapes, lemon, orange, papaya, parsley, buckwheat, plum, prune, rose hips, sweet peppers, tomato
- Food Sources of Vitamin E:
    - o Wheat germ oil, wheat germ, sunflower seeds, almonds
- Food Sources of Vitamin K:
    - o Eggs, avocado, banana, figs, abalone, asparagus, green beans, broccoli, brussel sprouts, carrot, cauliflower, escarole, kale, mustard greens, green peas, spinach

Minerals in Food Sources according to BodyBio Inc

- Food Sources of Potassium:
    - o Avocado, banana, cantaloupe, casaba melon, watermelon, potato, dates, grapefruit, orange, honeydew melon, lychee, orange, papaya, pineapple, prunes,

raisins, figs, milk, ricotta cheese, buckwheat, brown rice, dark rye, wheat germ clams, cod, mahi mahi, herring, lobster, salmon, red snapper, yellowtail, Cornish game hen, turkey, almonds, brazil nuts, cashews, coconut filberts, pecans, pistachio nuts, sesame seeds, sunflower seeds, walnuts, adzuki beans, kidney beans, lima beans, pinto beans, beets, broccoli, bok choy, Chinese cabbage, carrots, potato flour, soybeans, spinach, squash, Swiss chard

- Food Sources of Magnesium:
  - o Almonds, avocado, dates, prickly pear fruit, figs, apricots, buckwheat, wheat germ, brown rice, cashews, filberts, whole rye, pecans, macadamia nuts, sunflower seeds, soybeans, spinach, coconut, parsnips, sesame seeds
- Food Sources of Manganese:
  - o Mussels, escargot, clams, wheat germ, dark rye, coconut, pecans, pumpkin seeds, black walnuts, soybeans, almonds, sesame seeds, blackberries, loganberries, black cherries, pineapple, lima beans, potato flour, buckwheat, split peas, spinach
- Food Sources of Nitrogen Rich Foods:
  - o Protein containing foods as meat (beef, lamb, pork, sweetbreads, wild game), poultry (chicken, duck, turkey, Cornish hen, goose), eggs, dairy products (goat or cow's milk, soft cheese, feta cheese) and fish (Alaskan salmon, sardines, cod roe),

seeds, nuts, and legumes (soaked, very well cooked such as butter beans, lentils).

- Food Sources of Phosphorus:
  - o Pumpkin seeds, wheat germ, sunflower seeds, sesame seeds, cashews, cheese, eggs, buckwheat, brown rice, soybeans, millet, clams, crab, herring, mussels, salmon, sardines, scallops, beef, beef heart, duck, Cornish game hen, turkey, almonds, brazil nuts, pecans, black walnuts, navy beans, split peas
- Food Sources of Chromium:
  - o Papaya, onions, oysters, cantaloupe, fresh ground black pepper, brewer's yeast, organic liver, whole rye, eggs
- Food Sources of Iodine:
  - o Clams, shrimp, haddock, halibut, Alaskan salmon, sardines, eggs, seaweed
- Food Sources of Selenium:
  - o Seaweed, dark rye, wheat germ, brown rice, clams, lobster, red Swiss chard, butter trout, shrimp, scallops, cheddar cheese, cottage cheese, sunflower seeds, brazil nuts, cucumber
- Food Sources of Vanadium:
  - o Buckwheat, parsley, soybeans, eggs, and sunflower seeds
- Food Sources of Zinc:
  - o Oysters, ginger, beef, lamb, pecans, split peas, brazil nuts, egg yolk, dark rye, lima beans, feta cheese, rice polishings, wheat germ, crab, cashews, almonds, walnuts,

sunflower seeds, pumpkin seeds, hearts of palm, potato flour, garbanzo beans, chicken, mushrooms

- Food Sources of Calcium:
  - o Ricotta cheese, turnip greens, almonds, milk (cow, goat), canned Alaskan salmon, sardines, parsley, anchovies, bass, caviar, crab, lobster, brazil nuts, sesame seeds, pistachio, sunflower seeds, walnuts, great northern beans, kidney beans, navy beans, beet greens, broccoli, bok choy, Chinese cabbage, kale, soybeans, acorn squash, butternut squash, chestnuts, filberts, garbanzo beans
- Food Sources of Molybdenum:
  - o Buckwheat, wheat germ, lima beans, lentils, organic beef liver, beef heart, split peas, cauliflower, brown rice, eggs, dark rye, yams, green beans, sunflower seeds, garlic, spinach
- Food Sources of Copper:
  - o Buckwheat, clams, crab, lobster, oyster, organic beef liver, lamb liber, turkey-dark meat, almonds, brazil nuts, split peas, cashews, filberts, pecans, pistachio nuts, sesame seeds, sunflower seeds, walnuts, almonds
- Food Sources of Iron:
  - o Apricots, prunes, clams, mussels, organic beef, organic liver, beef heart, chicken, duck, almonds, brazil nuts, cashews, coconut, macadamia nuts, pistachio nuts,

pumpkin seeds, sesame seeds, sunflower seeds, black walnuts, kidney beans, lima beans, navy beans, white beans, refried pinto beans, lentils, snow peas, spinach, artichoke, millet, unsulfured prunes, lamb, eggs, parsley

Spectracell List of Vitamins & Minerals Correlated with Mental Health

ANXIETY

Chromium: Its effect on serotonin transmission may explain its anxiolytic (anxiety relieving) effect in animal studies.

Folate: Aids in production of neurotransmitters such as dopamine and serotonin which have a calming effect on mood.

Inositol: A neurochemical messenger in the brain, inositol (vitamin B8) affects dopamine and serotonin receptors; trials confirm it is very effective in reducing panic attacks.

Choline: Precursor to the neurotransmitter acetylcholine which affects focus and mood. Low levels of choline linked to anxiety.

Serine: Exerts a calming effect by buffering the adrenal response to physical or emotional stress. Lowered anxiety scores of patients with post-traumatic stress disorder.

Copper: Integral part of certain chemicals in the brain (such as endorphins) that calm anxious feelings. Anxiety-like behavior may be exacerbated with copper deficiency.

Magnesium: Regulated the HPA (hypothalamic-pituitary-adrenal) axis which controls physical and psychological reactions to stress; deficiency can induce anxiety and emotional hyper-reactivity.

Selenium: Repletion of selenium to normal levels reduced anxiety scores in clinical trials. Some suggest the mechanism of action is due its role in key regulatory proteins (selenoproteins).

Zinc: Reduces anxiety in clinical trials possibly due to its interaction with NMDA (N-methyl-D-aspartate) receptors in the brain which regulate mood.

Vitamin B6: Cofactor in synthesis of calming neurotransmitters such as GABA (gamma-amino butyric acid), serotonin and dopamine.

Vitamin B3: One of the symptoms of severe B3 deficiency (pellagra) is anxiety; pharmacological doses of B3 may enhance the calming effects of GABA in the brain; Converts tryptophan to serotonin.

Vitamins D & E: Low vitamin D status is linked to anxiety. Animal studies confirm the role of vitamins D and B in reducing anxiety-related behaviors.

Carnitine: Studies show that carnitine can reduce anxiety and improve feelings of well-being.

DEPRESSION

Magnesium: Deficiency damages NMDA (N-methyl-D-aspartate) receptors in the brain, which regulate mood; well-documented anti-depressant effects.

Selenium: Integral part of regulatory proteins (selenoproteins) in the brain; Supplementation trials are promising; May alleviate post-partum depression.

Chromium: Elevates serotonin (feel good neurotransmitter) levels in the brain. May be particularly effective on eating symptoms of depression such as carbohydrate craving and increased appetite due to its effect on blood sugar regulation.

Vitamin B12: Depression may be a manifestation of B12 deficiency. Repletion of B12 to adequate level scan improve treatment response; B12 deficiency common in psychiatric disorders.

Vitamin B6: Cofactor for serotonin and dopamine production (feel good chemicals). Studies indicate that low levels may predispose people to depression.

Vitamin B2: Low B2 has been implicated in depression due to its role in methylation reactions in the brain.

Vitamin D: Clinical trials suggest increasing blood levels of Vitamin D which is actually a hormone precursor; may improve symptoms of depression.

Carnitine: Increases serotonin and noradrenaline which lift mood. In trials, carnitine alleviates depression with few, if any, side effects.

Inositol: Influences signaling pathways in the brain. Particularly effective in SSRI (selective serotonin reuptake inhibitor) sensitive disorders.

Biotin: Part of the B-vitamin complex, biotin deficiency has induced depression in animal and human studies.

Antioxidants: Oxidative stress in the brain alters neurotransmitter function; Antioxidants protect our brain, which is very sensitive to oxidation; several antioxidants – Vitamins A, C and E, Lipoic Acid, CoQ10, Glutathione and Cysteine – play a key role in prevention and treatment of depression.

Serine: Regulates brain chemistry. Involved in NMDA receptor function; acts as a neurotransmitter. Low levels correlate with severity of depression.

Zinc: improves efficacy of antidepressant drugs. Useful for treatment resistant patients; regulates neurotransmitters.

FATIGUE

Carnitine: Transports fatty acids into mitochondria. Decreases both mental and physical fatigue in clinical trials.

Chromium: Promotes glucose uptake into cells, helping stabilize blood sugar.

Zinc: Deficiency lowers immunity and may cause muscle fatigue. Involved in several reactions for energy metabolism.

Asparagine: Supplementation of this amino acid delayed fatigue during exercise by decreasing the rate at which glycogen was used up; needed for gluconeogenesis, a process that allows glucose to be made from protein to prevent blood sugar from getting too low.

Biotin: Helps liver utilize glycogen for energy. Animal studies confirm that biotin deficiency causes clinical fatigue.

Glutamine: Mental and physical fatigue coincides with reduces levels of this amino acid various tissues. Supplementation makes muscle more sensitive to insulin, increasing energy levels.

Serine: Counteracts the overproduction of fatigue-causing stress hormones.

CoQ10: Deficiency causes fatigue due to its role in mitochondrial energy metabolism; therapeutic benefits particularly noticeable in chronic fatigue syndrome.

Fructose intolerance: Fatigue (and hypoglycemia) are classic symptoms of this condition since it depletes the main form of cellular energy, ATP.

Magnesium: Required to store energy molecule ATP; repletion of magnesium in chronic fatigue patients shows clinical improvement in energy levels.

Antioxidants: Several studies confirm that oxidative stress exacerbates clinical symptoms of fatigue. Mitochondrial dysfunction (inefficient energy metabolism) can be treated therapeutically with antioxidants such as Selenium, Cysteine, a-Lipoic acid and Glutathione, of which unusually low levels are seen in chronic fatigue patients.

Vitamin C: Assists iron uptake and transport; precursor to carnitine and several hormones that affect energy levels. Supplementation reduced fatigue in various trials.

Vitamin A: When cellular levels of Vitamin A are low

Vitamin E: Inverse correlation exists between fatigue and vitamin E levels.

Vitamin D: Low levels are seen

B Vitamins: Necessary for converting food into energy. Cofactors in the mitochondrial respiratory chain include B1, B2, B3, B5, B6, B12 and folate.

INSOMNIA

Vitamin B1 (Thiamin): In clinical trials, supplementation of healthy individuals that had marginal B1 deficiency improved their sleep.

Vitamin B3 (Niacin): Increases REM sleep; improves both quality and quantity of sleep by converting tryptophan to serotonin.

Folate & Vitamin B6: Both are cofactors for several neurotransmitters in the brain such as serotonin and dopamine, many of which regulate sleep patterns.

Vitamin B12: Normalizes circadian rhythms (sleep wake cycles). Therapeutic benefits of B12 supplementation, both oral and intravenous, seen in studies.

Magnesium: Improving magnesium status is associated with better quality sleep; mimics the action of melatonin. Also alleviates insomnia due to restless leg syndrome.

Zinc & Copper: Both interact with NMDA (N-methyl-D-aspartate) receptors in the brain that regulate sleep. A higher zinc/ copper ratio is linked to longer sleep duration.

Oleic Acid: This fatty acid is a precursor of oleamide, which regulates our drive for sleep and tends to accumulate in the spinal fluid of sleep-deprived animals. Oleic acid also facilitates the absorption of Vitamin A.

Vitamin A: Studies suggest Vitamin A deficiency alters brainwaves in non-REM sleep causing sleep to be less restorative.

METHYLATION

Vitamin B3: Maintains proper methylation of genes that suppress tumor formation and growth.

Vitamin B6: Cofactor for the enzyme (serine hydroxyl methyl transferase) that transfers methyl units.

Vitamin B12: B12 is a key enzyme needed in the synthesis of S-Adenosyl methionine (SAMe) the body's most important methyl donor. Methionine synthase, an enzyme that catalyzes the methylation cycle is B12 dependent.

Folate: Methyl donor for many reactions in the body, including neurotransmitter synthesis and conversion of homocysteine to methionine. Precursor to SAMe; required for proper DNA synthesis.

Choline: A major source of methyl groups (methyl-donor); deficiency linked to DNA damage.

Serine: Important methyl donor, especially in the case of folate deficiency.

Glutathione: Deficiency impairs methylation reactions and hinders synthesis of the methyl donor SAMe.

Vitamin C: Deficiency alters methylation patterns in cancer cells. Also a cofactor for methylating enzymes.

Copper: Several key enzymes needed for methylation reactions are copper dependent.

Magnesium: its role in the methylation of genes that affect glucose metabolism may explain the link between magnesium deficiency and diabetes.

Selenium: Inhibits a methylating enzyme (DNA methyltransferase) in cancer genes, effectively turning them off; selenoproteins protect DNA and metabolize methionine.

Zinc: Deficiency can lower the ability to use methyl groups from methyl donors such as SAMe, thus causing global hypo-methylation of DNA.

Vitamin B2: Helps recycle folate into a usable methyl-donor form; Precursor to FAD (flavin adenine dinucleotide) which assists methylation reactions.

Drug-Induced Nutrient Depletions as Outlined by Spectracell

ANTACIDS/ ULCER MEDICATIONS

- Such as Pepcid, Tagamet, Zantac, Prevacid, Prilosec, Magnesium & aluminum antacids

Nutrient deficiencies they can cause: Vitamin B12, Folic Acid, Vitamin D, Calcium, Iron and Zinc

ANTIBIOTICS

- Such as Gentamycin, neomycin, streptomycin, cephalosporins, penicillins

Nutrient deficiencies they can cause: B Vitamins, Vitamin K

- Such as Tetracyclines

Nutrient deficiencies they can cause: Calcium, Magnesium, Iron, Vitamin B6, Zinc

CHOLESTEROL DRUGS

- Such as Lipitor, Cretor, Zocor and others

Nutrient deficiencies they can cause: Coenzyme Q10

ANTIDEPRESSANTS

- Such as Adapin, Aventyl, Elavil, Pamelor, major tranquilizers (Thorazine, Mellaril, Prolixin, Serentil & others)

Nutrient deficiencies they can cause: Coenzyme Q10, Vitamin B2

FEMALE HORMONES

- Such as Estrogen/ Hormone Replacement/ Oral Contraceptives

Nutrient deficiencies they can cause: Vitamin B6, Folic Acid, Vitamin B1, Vitamin B2, Vitamin B3, Vitamin B12, Vitamin C, Magnesium, Selenium, Zinc

ANTICONVULSANTS

- Such as Phenobarbital & barbituates

Nutrient deficiencies they can cause: Vitamin D, Calcium, Folic Acid

- Such as Dilatin, Tegretol, Mysoline

Nutrient deficiencies they can cause: Biotin

- Such as Depakane/ Depacon

Nutrient deficiencies they can cause: Carnitine, Vitamin B12, Vitamin B1, Vitamin K, Copper, Selenium, Zinc

ANTI-INFLAMMATORIES

- Such as Steroids, Prednisone, Medrol, Aristocort, Decadron

Nutrient deficiencies they can cause: Calcium, Vitamin D, Magnesium, Zinc, Vitamin C, Vitamin B6, Vitamin B12, Folic Acid, Selenium, Chromium

- Such as NSAIDS (Motrin, Aleve, Advil, ANaprox, Dolobid, Feldene, Naprosyn and others)

Nutrient deficiencies they can cause: Folic Acid

- Such as Aspirin & Salicylates

Nutrient deficiencies they can cause: Vitamin C, Calcium, Folic Acid, Iron, Vitamin B5

DIURETICS

- Such as Loop Diuretics (Lasix, Burnex, Edecrin), Thiazide Diuretics (HcTZ, Enduron, Diuril, Lozol, Zaroxolyn, Hygroton)

Nutrient deficiencies they can cause: Calcium, Magnesium, Vitamin B1, Vitamin B6, Vitamin C, Zinc, Coenzyme Q10, Potassium, Sodium

- Such as Potassium Sparing Diuretics

Nutrient deficiencies they can cause: Calcium, Folic Acid, Zinc

CARDIOVASCULAR DRUGS

- Such as Antihypertensives (Catapres, Aldormet)

Nutrient deficiencies they can cause: Coenzyme Q10, Vitamin B6, Zinc, Vitamin B1

- Such as ACE Inhibitors (Capoten, Vasotec, Monopril)

Nutrient deficiencies they can cause: Zinc

- Such as Beta Blockers (Inderal, Corgard, Lopressor and others)

Nutrient deficiencies they can cause: Coenzyme Q10

DIABETIC DRUGS

- Metformin

Nutrient deficiencies it can cause: Coenzyme Q10, Vitamin B12, Folic Acid

- Such as Sulfonylureas (Tolinase, Micronase, Glynase, DiaBeta)

Nutrient deficiencies they can cause: Coenzyme Q10

ANTIVIRAL AGENTS

- Such as Zidovudine (Retrovir, AZT & other related drugs)

Nutrient deficiencies they can cause: Carnitine, Copper, Zinc, Vitamin B12

- Such as Foscarnet

Nutrient deficiencies it can cause: Calcium, Magnesium, Potassium

MINDFULNESS

Mindfulness is the practice of being fully engaged in the moment. One can practice mindfulness while doing a routine activity such as washing dishes or standing on line, or practice mindfulness mediation in which the goal is to just focus on one object. Either way, the idea is that we are, much of the time, on "automatic pilot;" most of the activities we engage in, our thoughts and our reactions to things happen pretty automatically. During mindfulness practice, we try to "watch" our thoughts – observing them rather than being them. We try to experience non-judgmental awareness of what we are thinking and feeling, rather than trying to escape or avoid, accepting the moment just as it isl

One mindfulness exercise that I routinely teach my clients involves the simultaneous awareness of all their senses. Try this:

- Begin by sitting comfortable in a chair or couch. Let it support you completely.

- Feel the soles of your feet against the ground, and the ground against your feet. Immerse yourself fully in this feeling. This start the exercise with the intention of grounding.

- Now bring your attention to your breath. Breathing out of your nose if possible, inhale deeply from your diaphragm, filling up your chest and belly simultaneously with air and exhale.

- Bring your awareness back to your feet against the ground.

- Now we will begin what is referred to as the body scan. Starting with you full awareness of your feet against the ground, raise that awareness into your ankles, shins, calves. Now on to your knees, this and pelvis. Stop here and focus completely on what it feels like to sit against the couch or chair. Continue with your awareness up into your belly, up to your ribs, your chest, your shoulders, down your arms, into your hands. Notice the feeling of your hands against the texture of the chair or couch. Bring your awareness back up to your shoulders, your back your neck, into your face and your head. Notice any tension.

- Bring your awarenss back to your feet against the ground.

- Take another deep breath like the other one.

- Bring your awareness back to your feet against the ground.

- With your full body awareness, now notice your sense of sight. Look around the room you are in and notice one thing you never noticed before.

- Bring your awareness back to your feet against the ground.

- With the full awareness of your body and your sight, bring your awareness to your sense of smell. If you don't smell anything in particular, really notice the air against your nostrils and into your throat when you breathe in.

- Bring your awareness back to your feet against the ground.

- With the full awareness of your body, sight, and sense of smell, bring your awareness to your sense of hearing. Notice one sound that you did not notice before.

- Bring your awareness back to your feet against the ground.

- Just sit with this total awareness and focus on one object in front of you one-mindfully. You may be feeling very present right now, very much "in" your body. You may find yourself drifting in and out of thoughts. Just watch your thoughts as if they are clouds passing by in front of you. Don't cling to a thought, just let it pass. Identify it as a thought – for example, in your head, say to yourself literally what is happening such as "oh there is that thought about how I have a deadline tomorrow at work."

The idea with the practice of mindfulness is that you can do it anywhere, any time. You don't have to be sitting and meditating. You can be driving or talking to someone. You can be waiting in line at the drugstore or sitting on the subway. The more you engage in things mindfully, the less anxious you will feel and the less you will react to uncomfortable thoughts and feelings.

ABOUT THE AUTHOR

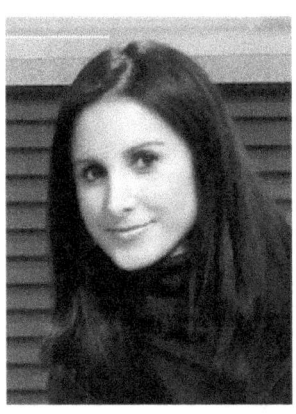

Dr. Niloo Dardashti is a Licensed Psychologist, Coach, and Board Certified Holistic Health Practitioner, living and practicing in New York City. She earned her Bachelor's in Science from New York University in 2000 and received additional training in Mindfulness, Meditation, and Reiki. In 2007, Dr. Dardashti received her doctorate in Clinical Psychology from Long Island University, with training in Cognitive Behavioral, Psychodynamic, Couples, Family, and Dialectical Behavior therapies.

After her graduate training, Dr. D. Niloo became certified in Herbology by the East West School of Herbology, where she received training in the medicinal use of foods and herbs. She then obtained training in targeted amino acid therapy for **mental health wellness and weight management** with both Julia Ross and Marty Hinz, two pioneers in the field. She is certified by Neuroscience Lab's Neuro Certification Program and board certified by the American Association of Drugless Practitioners.

In her private practice, Dr. D combines all of her training to provide coaching and therapy primarily with adults and couples. She is involved in various organizations and works with a network of professionals across the greater New York City metro area and provides trainings for other practitioners in Integrative Mental Health Treatment.

In 2011, Dr. D completed a documentary called "Into the Twilight Haze," which explores the "Twilight Phenomenon," the cross-generational female reaction to the Twilight books and movies, and provides insightful advice for relationships by various experts in the field of psychology. The film can be watched here: www.TwilightDocumentary.com or on Amazon.

Lastly, Dr. D will soon be releasing her new relationship self-help book titled "Fifty Shades of Women's Desires: The Allure of Twilight, Fifty Shades, and Other Pop-Culture Phenomena." This is a handbook to relationships for both men and women, uncovering and explaining the classic question: Is it me or the relationship? To learn more about Dr. D you can visit www.DrNilooDardashti.com

References

DEPRESSION

1. **Role of omega-3 fatty acids in the treatment of depressive disorders: a comprehensive meta-analysis of randomized clinical trials.**
   - http://www.ncbi.nlm.nih.gov/pubmed/24805797
     - PMID: 24805797
     - Grosso G[1], Pajak A[2], Marventano S[3], Castellano S[1], Galvano F[1], Bucolo C[1], Drago F[1], Caraci F[4].
     - PLoS One. 2014 May 7;9(5):e96905. doi: 10.1371/journal.pone.0096905. eCollection 2014.

2. **A comparative study of efficacy of l-5-hydroxytryptophan and fluoxetine in patients presenting with first depressive episode.**
   - http://www.ncbi.nlm.nih.gov/pubmed/23380314
     - PMID: 23380314
     - Jangid P[1], Malik P, Singh P, Sharma M, Gulia AK.
     - Asian J Psychiatr. 2013 Feb;6(1):29-34. doi: 10.1016/j.ajp.2012.05.011. Epub 2012 Jul 12.

3. **The treatment of depression with L-5-hydroxytryptophan versus imipramine. Results of two open and one double-blind study.**
   - Angst J, Woggon B, Schoepf J.
   - *Arch Psychiatr Nervenkr.* 1977;224:175–186.

4. **5-Hydroxytryptophan: A clinically effective serotonin precursor.**
   - Birdsall TC.
   - *Altern Med Rev.*1998;3:271–280.

5. **5-hydroxytryptophan: a review of its antidepressant efficacy and adverse effects.**
   - Byerley WF, Judd LL, Reimherr FW, et al.
   - *J Clin Psychopharmacol.* 1987;7:127-137.

6. **A functional-dimensional approach to depression: Serotonin deficiency as a target syndrome in a comparison of 5-hydroxytryptophan and fluvoxamine.**
   - Poldinger W, Calanchini B, Schwarz W.
   - *Psychopathology.* 1991;24:53-81.

7. **Effect of a serotonin precursor and uptake inhibitor in anxiety disorders; a double-blind comparison of 5-hydroxytryptophan, clomipramine and placebo.**
   - Kahn RS, Westenberg HG, Verhoeven WM, et al.
   - *Int Clin Psychopharmacol.* 1987;2:33-45.

8. **A functional-dimensional approach to depression: Serotonin deficiency as a target syndrome in a comparison of 5-hydroxytryptophan and fluvoxamine.**
   - Poldinger W, Calanchini B, Schwarz W.
   - *Psychopathology.* 1991;24:53-81.
     - ➢ *ABSTRACT:*
     - ➢ A 6-week study of 63 people given either 5-HTP (100 mg 3 times daily) or an antidepressant in the Prozac family (fluvoxamine, 50 mg 3 times daily). 17 Researchers found equal benefit between the supplement and the drug. However, 5-HTP caused fewer and less severe side effects.

9. **Use of neurotransmitter precursors for treatment of depression.**
- Meyers S.
- *Altern Med Rev.* 2000;5(1):64-71.

10. **Nutrient intakes and the common mental disorders in women.**
- http://www.ncbi.nlm.nih.gov/ pubmed/22397891
  - PMID: 22397891
  - Jacka FN[1], Maes M, Pasco JA, Williams LJ, Berk M.
  - J Affect Disord. 2012 Dec 1;141(1):79-85. doi: 10.1016/j.jad.2012.02.018. Epub 2012 Mar 6.

11. **Phenylalanine for Endogenous Depression**
- http://www.orthomolecular. com/?ctr=article&act=show&id=17
  - A. Yaryura-Tobias, B. Heller, H. Spatz, and E. Fischer

12. **Oral S-adenosyl-L-methionine In Depression**
- http://www.sciencedirect.com/science/ article/pii/S0011393X05804242
  - M. De Vanna, R. Rigamonti

13. **The Treatment of Depression in General Practice: A Comparison of L-tryptophan, Amitriptyline, and a Combination of L-tryptophan and Amitriptyline with Placebo.**
    - http://www.ncbi.nlm.nih.gov/pubmed/7156248
        - PMID: 7156248
        - Thomson J, Rankin H, Ashcroft GW, Yates CM, McQueen JK, Cummings SW.
        - Psychol Med. 1982 Nov;12(4):741-51.

14. **Tyrosine for the Treatment of Depression.**
    - http://www.ncbi.nlm.nih.gov/pubmed/6443584
        - PMID: 6443584
        - Gelenberg AJ, Gibson CJ.
        - Nutr Health. 1984;3(3):163-73.

15. **DL-phenylalanine Versus Imipramine: A Double-Blind Controlled Study.**
    - http://www.ncbi.nlm.nih.gov/pubmed/387000
        - PMID: 387000
        - Beckmann H, Athen D, Olteanu M, Zimmer R.
        - Arch Psychiatr Nervenkr. 1979 Jul 4;227(1):49-58.

16. **Folic Acid Deficiency and Depression**
- http://www.ncbi.nlm.nih.gov/ pubmed/7433596
  - PMID: 7433596
  - Ghadirian AM, Ananth J, Engelsmann F.
  - Psychosomatics. 1980 Nov;21(11):926-9.

ADHD

17. **The effects of L-theanine (Suntheanine®) on objective sleep quality in boys with attention deficit hyperactivity disorder (ADHD): a randomized, double blind, placebo-controlled clinical trial.**
- http://www.ncbi.nlm.nih.gov/ pubmed/22214254
  - PMID: 22214254
  - Lyon MR[1], Kapoor MP, Juneja LR.
  - Altern Med Rev. 2011 Dec;16(4):348-54.

18. **Ginkgo biloba treating patients with attention-deficit disorder.**
- http://www.ncbi.nlm.nih.gov/ pubmed/19441138
  - PMID: 19441138
  - Niederhofer H.
  - Phytother Res. 2010 Jan;24(1):26-7. doi: 10.1002/ptr.2854.

19. **Panax ginseng may improve some symptoms of attention-deficit hyperactivity disorder.**
    - http://www.ncbi.nlm.nih.gov/pubmed/22435351
      - PMID: 22435351
      - Niederhofer H.
      - J Diet Suppl. 2009;6(1):22-7. doi: 10.1080/19390210802687221.

20. **Urinary catecholamines in children with attention deficit hyperactivity disorder (ADHD): modulation by a polyphenolic extract from pine bark (pycnogenol).**
    - http://www.ncbi.nlm.nih.gov/pubmed/18019397
      - PMID: 18019397
      - Dvoráková M[1], Jezová D, Blazícek P, Trebatická J, Skodácek I, Suba J, Iveta W, Rohdewald P, Duracková Z.
      - Nutr Neurosci. 2007 Jun-Aug; 10(3-4):151-7.

21. **Role of iron in the treatment of attention deficit-hyperactivity disorder.**
    - http://www.ncbi.nlm.nih.gov/pubmed/23582950
      - PMID: 23582950
      - Soto-Insuga V[1], Calleja ML, Prados M, Castaño C, Losada R, Ruiz-Falcó ML.
      - An Pediatr (Barc). 2013 Oct;79(4):230-5. doi: 10.1016/j.anpedi.2013.02.008. Epub 2013 Apr 11.

22. **Treatment of attention deficit hyperactivity disorder with monoamine amino acid precursors and organic cation transporter assay interpretation**
   - http://www.ncbi.nlm.nih.gov/pmc/articles/PMC3035600/
     - Marty Hinz, Alvin Stein, [...], and Thomas Uncini

SLEEP

23. **Treatment of insomnia: an alternative approach.**
   - Attele AS, Xie JT, Yuan CS. *Altern Med Rev.* 2000;5(3):249-259.

24. **Human sleep and 5-HTP. Effects of repeated high doses and of association with benserazide (RO.04.4602).**
   - http://www.ncbi.nlm.nih.gov/pubmed/60227
     - PMID: 60227
     - Autret A, Minz M, Bussel B, Cathala HP, Castaigne P.
     - Electroencephalogr Clin Neurophysiol. 1976 Oct; 41(4): 408-13.

25. **The effect of melatonin, magnesium, and zinc on primary insomnia in long-term care facility residents in Italy: a double blind, placebo-controlled clinical trial.**
   - http://www.ncbi.nlm.nih.gov/pubmed/21226679

- PMID: 21226679
- Rondanelli M[1], Opizzi A, Monteferrario F, Antoniello N, Manni R, Klersy C.
- J Am Geriatr Soc. 2011 Jan;59(1):82-90. doi: 10.1111/j.1532-5415.2010.03232.x.

26. **The Effect of L-Tryptophan on Daytime Sleep Latency in Normals: Correlation With Blood Levels**
  - http://www.journalsleep.org/ViewAbstract. aspx?pid=25050
    - C.F.P. George, T.W. Millar, P.J. Hanly and M.H. Kryger
    - *Section of Respiratory Medicine, University of Manitoba, Winnipeg, Manitoba, Canada*

27. **Evaluation of L-Tryptophan for treatment of insomnia: a review.**
  - http://www.ncbi.nlm.nih.gov/pubmed/3090582
    - PMID: 3090582
    - Schneider-Helmert D, Spinweber CL.

MOOD

28. **Efficacy of vitamin B-6 in the treatment of premenstrual syndrome: systematic review**
  - http://www.ncbi.nlm.nih.gov/pmc/articles/ PMC27878/
    - Katrina M Wyatt, non-clinical lecturer in reproductive endocrinology, Paul W Dimmock, researcher, [...], and P M Shaughn O'Brien, professor

➢ **CONCLUSIONS:**
➢ Conclusions are limited by the low quality of most of the trials included. Results suggest that doses of vitamin B-6 up to 100 mg/day are likely to be of benefit in treating premenstrual symptoms and premenstrual depression.

29. **The Impact of Selenium Supplementation on Mood**
   - http://www.ncbi.nlm.nih.gov/pubmed/1873372
     - PMID: 1873372
     - Benton D[1], Cook R.
     - Biol Psychiatry. 1991 Jun 1;29(11):1092-8.

30. **Vitamin Supplementation For 1 Year Improves Mood**
   - http://www.ncbi.nlm.nih.gov/pubmed/7477807
     - PMID: 7477807
     - Benton D[1], Haller J, Fordy J.
     - Neuropsychobiology. 1995;32(2):98-105.
       ➢ **ABSTRACT:**
       ➢ ....These changes in mood after a year occurred even though the blood status of 9 vitamins reached a plateau after 3 months: this improvement in mood was associated in particular with improved riboflavin and pyridoxine status. In females baseline thiamin

status was associated with poor mood and an improvement in thiamin status after 3 months was associated with improved mood.

31. **Vitamins, Minerals, and Mood**
   - Kaplan B., Field C., Crawford S., Simpson J.

OTHER:

32. **Treatment of pediatric restless legs syndrome.**
   - http://www.ncbi.nlm.nih.gov/pubmed/24198314
      - PMID: 24198314
      - Amos LB[1], Grekowicz ML, Kuhn EM, Olstad JD, Collins MM, Norins NA, D'Andrea LA.
      - Clin Pediatr (Phila). 2014 Apr;53(4):331-6. doi: 10.1177/0009922813507997. Epub 2013 Nov 6.

33. **A prospective, randomized double blind, placebo-controlled study of safety and efficacy of a high-concentration full-spectrum extract of Ashwagandha root in reducing stress and anxiety in adults.**
   - http://www.ncbi.nlm.nih.gov/pubmed/23439798
      - PMID: 23439798
      - Chandrasekhar K[1], Kapoor J, Anishetty S.
      - Indian J Psychol Med. 2012 Jul;34(3):255-62. doi: 10.4103/0253-7176.106022.

34. Influence of Withania somnifera on obsessive-compulsive disorder in mice.
- http://www.ncbi.nlm.nih.gov/pubmed/22546655
  - PMID: 22546655
  - Kaurav BP[1], Wanjari MM, Chandekar A, Chauhan NS, Upmanyu N.
  - Asian Pac J Trop Med. 2012 May;5(5):380-4. doi: 10.1016/S1995-7645(12)60063-7.

35. The Effect of L-tryptophan on Seasonal Affective Disorder
- http://www.ncbi.nlm.nih.gov/pubmed/2182615
  - PMID: 2182615
  - McGrath RE[1], Buckwald B, Resnick EV.
  - J Clin Psychiatry. 1990 Apr;51(4):162-3.

ASPARTAME

36. Neurobehavioral Effects of Aspartame Consumption
- http://www.ncbi.nlm.nih.gov/pubmed/24700203
  - PMID: 24700203
  - Lindseth GN[1], Coolahan SE, Petros TV, Lindseth PD.
  - Res Nurs Health. 2014 Jun;37(3):185-93. doi: 10.1002/nur.21595. Epub 2014 Apr 3.

37. **The Effect of Aspartame Metabolites on Human Erythrocyte Membrane Acetylcholinesterase Activity.**
   - http://www.ncbi.nlm.nih.gov/pubmed/16129618
     - PMID: 16129618
     - Tsakiris S[1], Giannoulia-Karantana A, Simintzi I, Schulpis KH.
     - Pharmacol Res. 2006 Jan;53(1):1-5. Epub 2005 Aug 29.

38. **Aspartame Ingestion and Headaches: A Randomized Crossover Trial.**
   - http://www.ncbi.nlm.nih.gov/pubmed/7936222
     - PMID: 7936222
     - Van den Eeden SK[1], Koepsell TD, Longstreth WT Jr, van Belle G, Daling JR, McKnight B.
     - Neurology. 1994 Oct;44(10):1787-93.

39. **Migraine MLT-Down: An Unusual Presentation of Migraine in Patients with Aspartame-Triggered Headaches.**
   - http://www.ncbi.nlm.nih.gov/pubmed/11703479
     - PMID: 11703479
     - Newman LC[1], Lipton RB.
     - Headache. 2001 Oct;41(9):899-901.